The Vibrant Guidebo
Recipe

Boost Your Metabolism and Enjoy Your Meals with Incredibly
Easy Recipes

Lola Rogers

Table of contents

Delicious Garlic Tomatoes

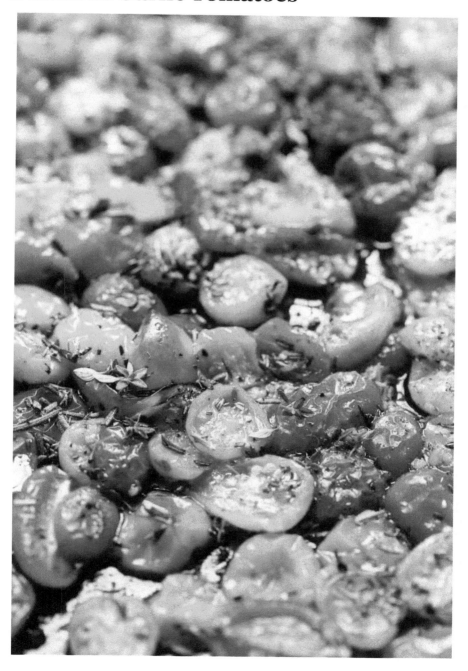

Serving: 4

Prep Time: 10 minutes

Cook Time: 50 minutes

Ingredients:

- 4 garlic cloves, crushed
- 1 pound mixed cherry tomatoes
- 3 thyme sprigs, chopped
- Pinch of sunflower seeds
- Black pepper as needed
- ¼ cup olive oil

How To:

1. Preheat your oven to 325 degrees F.
2. Take a baking dish and add tomatoes, olive oil and thyme.
3. Season with sunflower seeds and pepper and mix.
4. Bake for 50 minutes.
5. Divide tomatoes and pan juices and serve.
6. Enjoy!

Nutrition (Per Serving)

Calories: 100

Fat: 0g

Carbohydrates: 1g

Protein: 6g

Mashed Celeriac

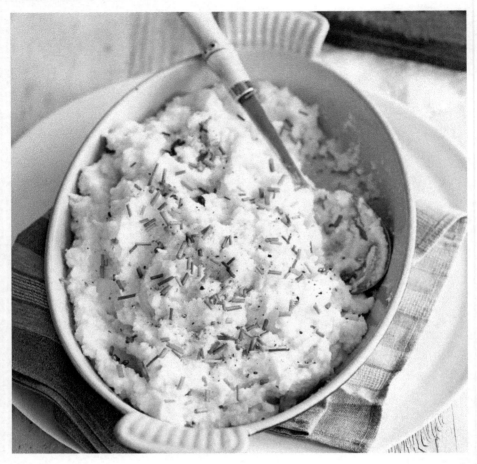

Serving: 4

Prep Time: 10 minutes

Cook Time: 20 minutes

Ingredients:

- 2 celeriac, washed, peeled and diced
- 2 teaspoons extra-virgin olive oil
- 1 tablespoon honey
- ½ teaspoon ground nutmeg
- Sunflower seeds and pepper as needed

How To:

1. Pre-heat your oven to 400 degrees F.

2. Line a baking sheet with aluminum foil and keep it on the side.

3. Take a large bowl and toss celeriac and olive oil.

4. Spread celeriac evenly on a baking sheet.

5. Roast for 20 minutes until tender.

6. Transfer to a large bowl.

7. Add honey and nutmeg.

8. Use a potato masher to mash the mixture until fluffy.

9. Season with sunflower seeds and pepper.

10. Serve and enjoy!

Nutrition (Per Serving)

Calories: 136

Fat: 3g

Carbohydrates: 26g

Protein: 4g

Spicy Wasabi Mayonnaise

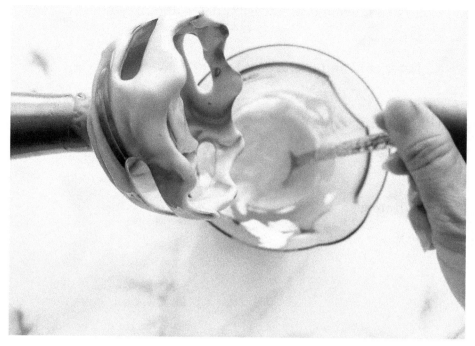

Serving: 4

Prep Time: 15 minutes

Cook Time: Nil

Ingredients:

- 1 cup mayonnaise
- ½ tablespoon wasabi paste

How To:

1.   Take a bowl and mix wasabi paste and mayonnaise.

2.   Mix well.

3.   Let it chill and use as needed.

Nutrition (Per Serving)

Calories: 388

Fat: 42g

Carbohydrates: 1g

Protein: 1g

Mediterranean Kale Dish

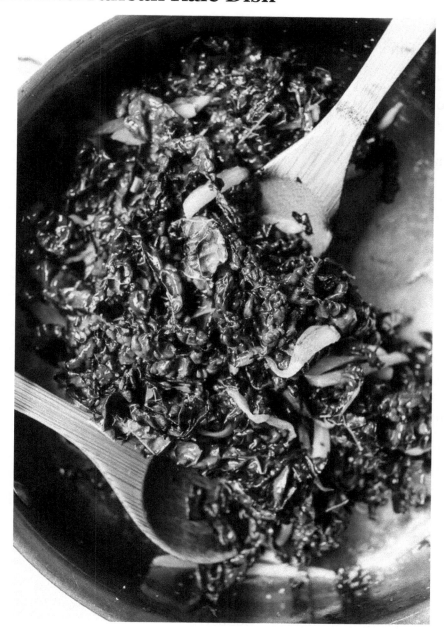

Serving: 6

Prep Time: 15 minutes

Cook Time: 10 minutes

Ingredients:

- 12 cups kale, chopped
- 2 tablespoons lemon juice
- 1 tablespoon olive oil
- 1 teaspoon coconut aminos
- Sunflower seeds and pepper as needed

How To:

1.   Add a steamer insert to your saucepan.

2.   Fill the saucepan with water up to the bottom of the steamer.

3.   Cover and bring water to boil (medium-high heat).

4.   Add kale to the insert and steam for 7-8 minutes.

5.   Take a large bowl and add lemon juice, olive oil, sunflower seeds, coconut aminos, and pepper.

6.   Mix well and add the steamed kale to the bowl.

7.   Toss and serve.

8.   Enjoy!

Nutrition (Per Serving)

Calories: 350

Fat: 17g

Carbohydrates: 41g

Protein: 11g

Spicy Kale Chips

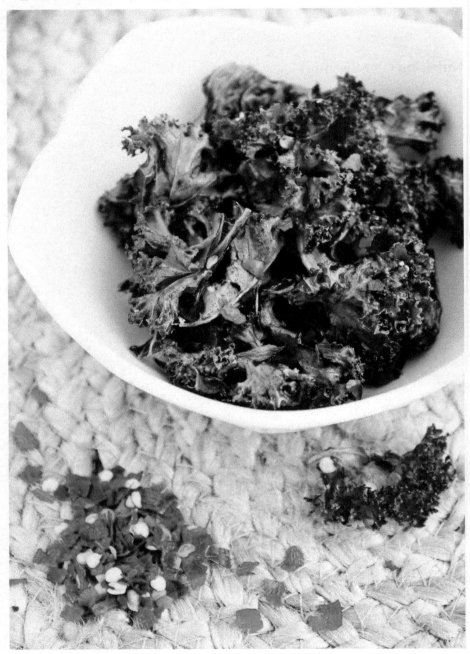

Serving: 4

Prep Time: 10 minutes

Cook Time: 25 minutes

Ingredients:

- 3 cups kale, stemmed and thoroughly washed, torn in 2-inch pieces
- 1 tablespoon extra-virgin olive oil
- ½ teaspoon chili powder
- ¼ teaspoon sea sunflower seeds

How To:

1. Pre-heat your oven to 300 degrees F.
2. Line 2 baking sheets with parchment paper and keep it on the side.
3. Dry kale entirely and transfer to a large bowl.
4. Add olive oil and toss.
5. Make sure each leaf is covered.

6. Season kale with chili powder and sunflower seeds, toss again.

7. Divide kale between baking sheets and spread into a single layer.

8. Bake for 25 minutes until crispy.

9. Cool the chips for 5 minutes and serve.

10. Enjoy!

Nutrition (Per Serving)

Calories: 56

Fat: 4g

Carbohydrates: 5g

Protein: 2g

Fudge Brownies

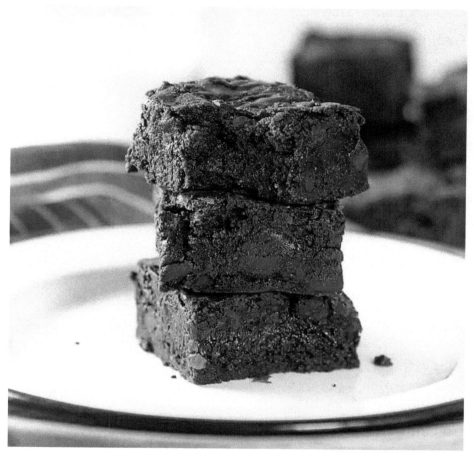

Nutritional Facts

servings per container   9

Prep Total   10 min

Serving Size 2/3 cup (70g)

Amount per serving 10

Calories

% Daily Value

Total Fat 20g   2%

Saturated Fat 2g   10%

Trans Fat 4g -

Cholesterol   10%

Sodium 50mg   12%

Total Carbohydrate 7g   20%

Dietary Fiber 4g   7%

Total Sugar 12g   -

Protein 3g

Vitamin C 2mcg   19%

Calcium 260mg   20%

Iron 8mg   8%

Potassium 235mg   6%

Ingredients

Instructions:

1.   Preheat oven to 350°F and grease a 9 x 13-inch baking pan.

2.   Add dry ingredients in a mixing bowl. Whisk together wet ingredients and fold into the dry ingredients.

3.   If desired, add half the chocolate chips and chopped walnuts to the mix. Pour mixture into the prepared pan and sprinkle with remaining chocolate chips and walnuts, if using.

4.   For fudge-like brownies, bake for 20-25 minutes. For cake-like brownies, bake 25-30 minutes. Let the brownies cool slightly before serving.

Pomegranate Quinoa Porridge

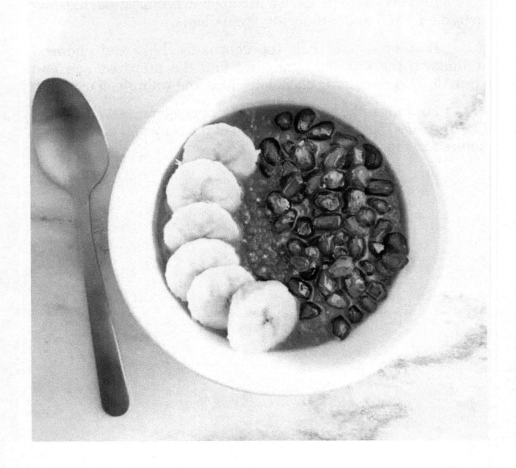

Nutritional Facts

servings per container   4

Prep Total   10 min

Serving Size 2/3 cup (40g)

Amount per serving 22

Calories

% Daily Value

Total Fat 12g 20%

Saturated Fat 2g   4%

Trans Fat 01g   1.22%

Cholesterol   22%

Sodium 170mg   10%

Total Carbohydrate 34g   22%

Dietary Fiber 5g   14%

Total Sugar 7g   -

Protein 3g

Vitamin C 2mcg   10%

Calcium 260mg   20%

Iron 0mg   40%

Potassium 235mg   6%

Ingredients

- 1 1/2 cup quinoa flakes
- 2 1/2 teaspoons cinnamon
- 1 teaspoon vanilla extract

- 10 organic pDashes, pitted and cut into 1/4's

- 1 pomegranate pulp

- 1/4 cup desiccated coconut

- Stewed apples

- Coconut flakes to garnish

Instructions:

1. Gently place quinoa & almond milk into saucepan, & stir on medium to low heat for 9 minutes, until it smooth

2. Include cinnamon, desiccated coconut & vanilla extract & taste

3. Pit pDashes & cut into quarters include to porridge stir in well

4. Serve into individual bowls

5. Add a scoop of stewed apple (kindly view recipe below), pomegranates, pDashes & coconut flakes

6. Ready to eat!

Stewed apples

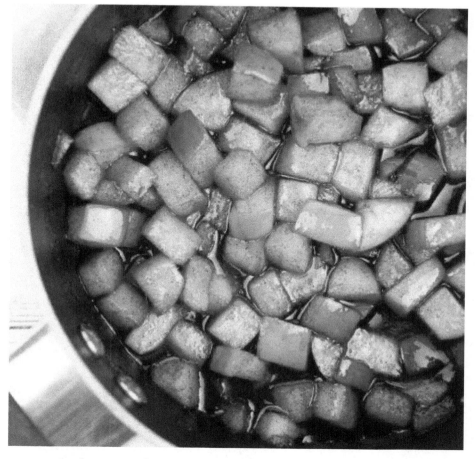

1. Peel, core, slice apples and place into a saucepan with water

2. Cook apples on medium heat, until extremely soft

3. Remove from heat, drain & mash apples

4. Ready to serve and enjoy your breakfast!

Cinnamon and Coconut Porridge

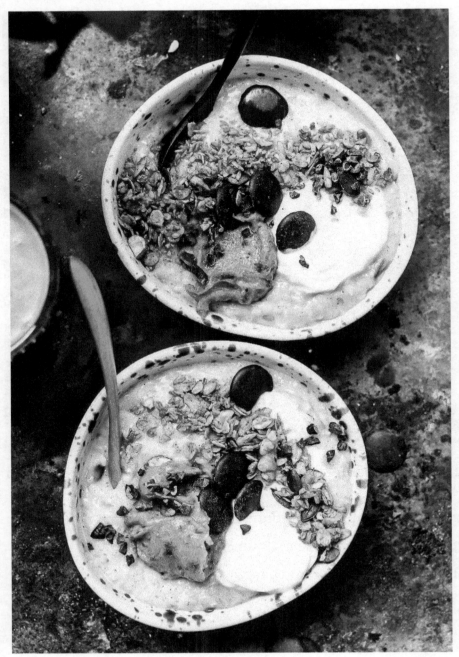

Serving: 4

Prep Time: 5 minutes

Cook Time: 5 minutes

Ingredients:

- 1 cup water
- 1/2 cup 36-percent low-fat cream
- ½ cup unsweetened dried coconut, shredded
- 1 tablespoon oat bran
- 1 tablespoon flaxseed meal
- 1/2 tablespoon almond butter
- 1 ½ teaspoons stevia
- ½ teaspoon cinnamon
- Toppings, such as blueberries or banana slices

How To:

1.   Add the ingredients to alittle pot and blend well until fully incorporated

2.   Transfer the pot to your stove over medium-low heat and convey the combination to a slow boil.

3.   Stir well and take away from the warmth .

4.   Divide the mixture into equal servings and allow them to sit for 10 minutes.

5.   Top together with your desired toppings and enjoy!

Nutrition (Per Serving)

Calories: 171

Fat: 16g

Protein: 2g

Carbohydrates: 8g

Coconut Porridge

Serving: 2

Prep Time: 15 minutes

Cook Time: Nil

Ingredients:

- 2 tablespoons coconut flour
- 2 tablespoons vanilla protein powder
- 3 tablespoons Golden Flaxseed meal
- 1 ½ cups almond milk, unsweetened
- Powdered Erythritol

How To:

1.   Take a bowl and blend within the flaxseed meal, protein powder, coconut flour and blend well.

2.   Add the combination to the saucepan (placed over medium heat).

3.   Add almond milk and stir, let the mixture thicken.

4.   Add your required amount of sweetener and serve.

5.   Enjoy!

Nutrition (Per Serving)

Calories: 259

Fat: 13g

Carbohydrates: 5g

Protein: 16g

Classic Apple and Cinnamon Oatmeal

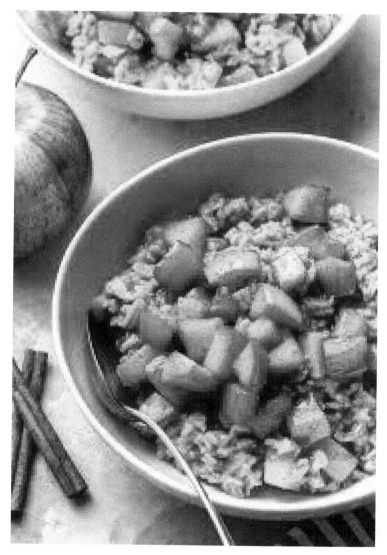

Serving: 4

Prep Time: 15 minutes

Cook Time: 7-9 hours

Ingredients:

- 1 apple, cored, peeled and diced
- 1 cup steel-cut oats
- 2 ½ cups unsweetened vanilla almond milk
- 2 tablespoons honey
- ½ teaspoon vanilla extract
- 1 teaspoon ground cinnamon

How To:

1. Grease the Slow Cooker well.
2. Add the listed ingredients to your Slow Cooker and stir.
3. Cover with lid and cook on LOW for 7-9 hours.
4. Serve and enjoy!

Nutrition (Per Serving)

Calories: 126

Fat: 3g

Carbohydrates: 25g

Protein: 3g

Carrot and Zucchini Oatmeal

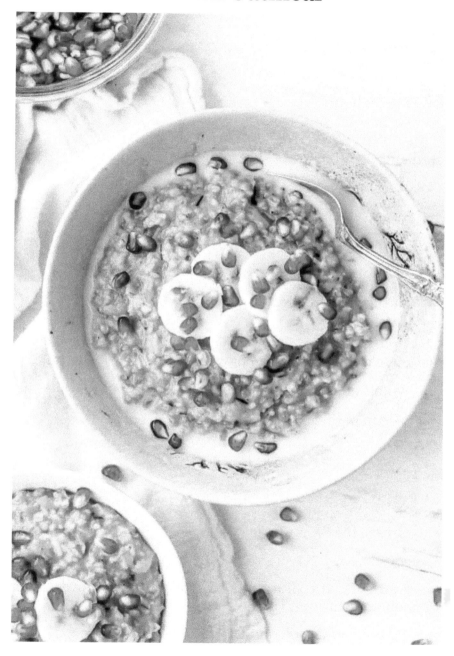

Serving: 3

Prep Time: 10 minutes

Cook Time: 8 hours

Ingredients:

- ½ cup steel cut oats
- 1 cup coconut milk
- 1 carrot, grated
- ¼ zucchini, grated
- Pinch of nutmeg
- ½ teaspoon cinnamon powder
- 2 tablespoons brown sugar
- ¼ cup pecans, chopped

How To:

1.   Grease the Slow Cooker well.

2.   Add oats, zucchini, milk, carrot, nutmeg, cloves, sugar, cinnamon and stir well.

3.   Place lid and cook on LOW for 8 hours.

4. Divide amongst serving bowls and enjoy!

Nutrition (Per Serving)

Calories: 200

Fat: 4g

Carbohydrates: 11g

Protein: 5g

Blueberry and Walnut "Steel" Oatmeal

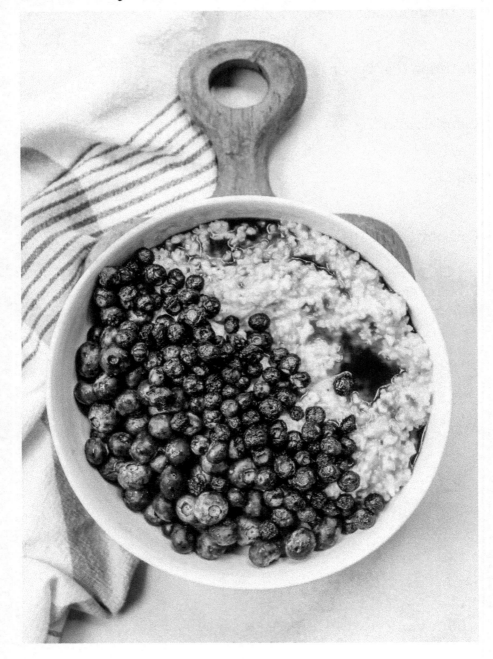

Serving: 8

Prep Time: 5 minutes

Cook Time: 7-8 hours

Ingredients:

- 2 cups steel-cut oats
- 6 cups water
- 2 cups low-fat milk
- 2 cups fresh blueberries
- 1 ripe banana, mashed
- 1 teaspoon vanilla extract
- 2 teaspoons ground cinnamon
- 2 tablespoons brown sugar
- Pinch of salt
- ½ cup walnuts, chopped

How To:

1.   Grease the within of your Slow Cooker.

2.   Add oats, milk, water, blueberries, banana, vanilla, sugar , cinnamon and salt to your Slow Cooker.

3.   Stir.

4.   Place lid and cook on LOW for 7-8 hours.

5.   Serve warm with a garnish of chopped walnuts.

6.   Enjoy!

Nutrition (Per Serving)

Calories: 372

Fat: 14g

Carbohydrates: 56g

Protein: 8g

Shrimp and Egg Medley

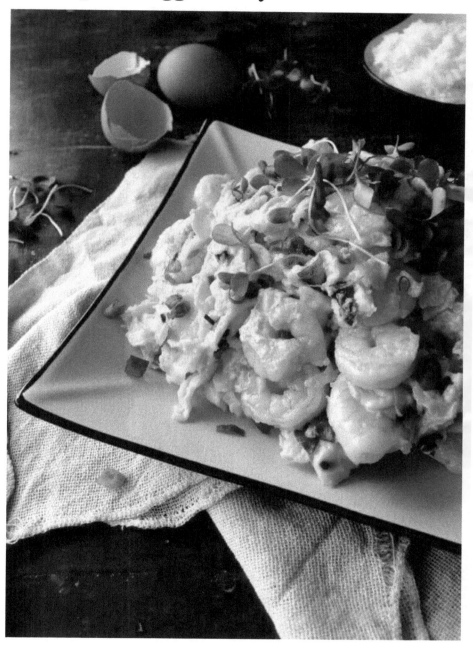

Serving: 4

Prep Time: 15 minutes

Cook Time: nil

Ingredients:

- 4 hardboiled eggs, peeled and chopped
- 1-pound cooked shrimp, peeled and de-veined, chopped
- 1 sprig fresh dill, chopped
- ¼ cup mayonnaise
- 1 teaspoon Dijon mustard
- 4 fresh lettuce leaves

How To:

1. Take an outsized serving bowl and add the listed ingredients (except lettuce.)
2. Stir well.
3. Serve over bet of lettuce leaves.
4. Enjoy!

Nutrition (Per Serving)

Calories: 292

Fat: 17g

Carbohydrates: 1.6g

Protein: 30g

Crispy Walnut Crumbles

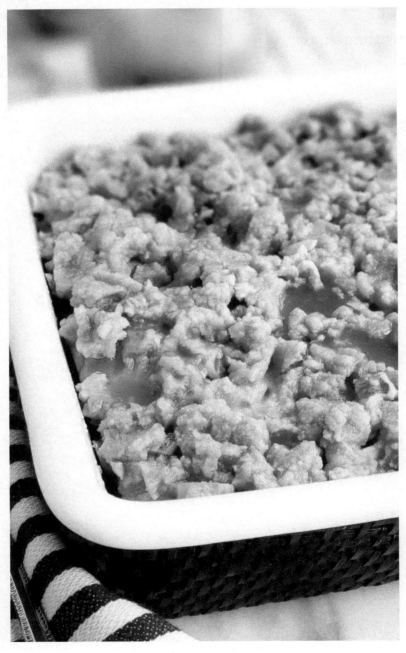

Serving: 10

Prep Time: 10 minutes

Cook Time: 8 minutes

Ingredients:

- 6 ounces kite ricotta/cashew cheese, grated
- 2 tablespoons walnuts, chopped
- 1 tablespoon almond butter
- ½ tablespoon fresh thyme chopped

How To:

1. Preheat your oven to 350 degrees F.

2. Take two large rimmed baking sheets and line with parchment.

3. Add cheese, almond butter to a kitchen appliance and blend.

4. Add walnuts to the combination and pulse.

5. Take a tablespoon and scoop mix onto a baking sheet.

6. Top them with chopped thymes.

7. Bake for 8 minutes, transfer to a cooling rack.

8. Let it cool for half-hour .

9.   Serve and enjoy!

Nutrition (Per Serving)

Calories: 80

Fat: 3g

Carbohydrates: 7g

Protein: 7g

Duck with Cucumber and Carrots

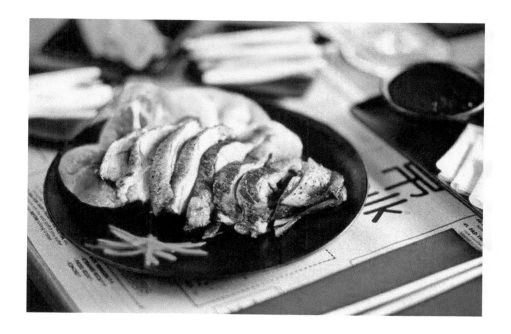

Serving: 8

Prep Time: 10 minutes

Cook Time: 40 minutes

Ingredients:

- 1 duck, cut up into medium pieces
- 1 chopped cucumber, chopped

- 1 tablespoon low sodium vegetable stock
- 2 carrots, chopped
- 2 cups of water
- Black pepper as needed
- 1-inch ginger piece, grated

How To:

1. Add duck pieces to your Instant Pot.

2. Add cucumber, stock, carrots, water, ginger, pepper and stir.

3. Lock up the lid and cook on low for 40 minutes.

4. Release the pressure naturally.

5. Serve and enjoy!

Nutrition (Per Serving)

Calories: 206

Fats: 7g

Carbs: 28g

Protein: 16g

Parmesan Baked Chicken

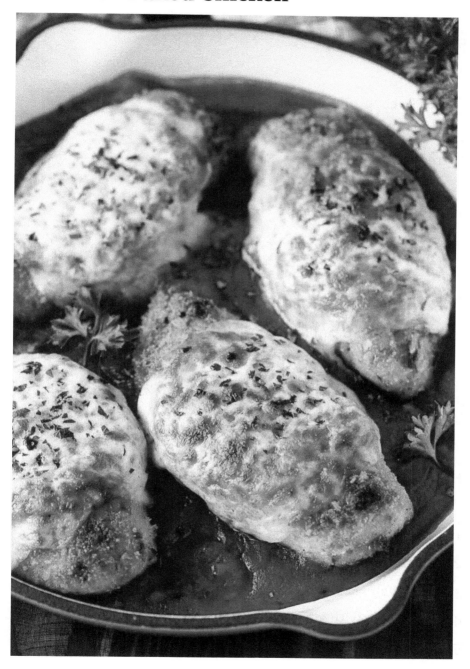

Serving: 2

Prep Time: 5 minutes

Cook Time: 20 minutes

Ingredients:

- 2 tablespoons ghee
- 2 boneless chicken breasts, skinless
- Pink sunflower seeds
- Freshly ground black pepper
- ½ cup mayonnaise, low fat
- ¼ cup parmesan cheese, grated
- 1 tablespoon dried Italian seasoning, low fat, low sodium
- ¼ cup crushed pork rinds

How To:

1. Preheat your oven to 425 degrees F.
2. Take an outsized baking dish and coat with ghee.
3. Pat chicken breasts dry and wrap with a towel.
4. Season with sunflower seeds and pepper.
5. Place in baking dish.

6.   Take alittle bowl and add mayonnaise, parmesan cheese, Italian seasoning.

7.   Slather mayo mix evenly over pigeon breast .

8.   Sprinkle crushed pork rinds on top.

9.   Bake for 20 minutes until topping is browned.

10.   Serve and enjoy!

Nutrition (Per Serving)

Calories: 850

Fat: 67g

Carbohydrates: 2g

Protein: 60g

Buffalo Chicken Lettuce Wraps

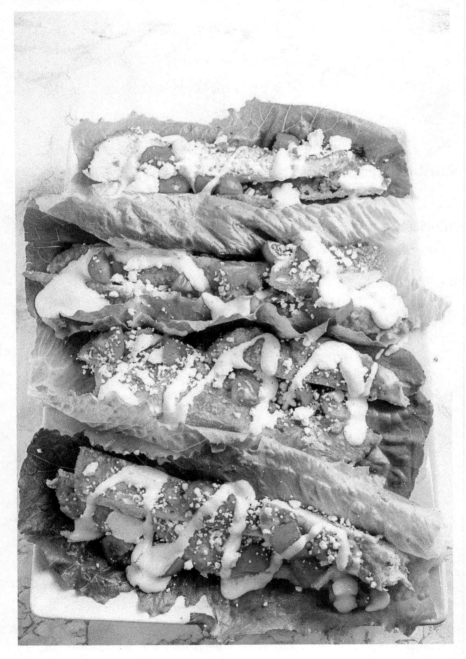

Serving: 2

Prep Time: 35 minutes

Cook Time: 10 minutes

Ingredients:

- 3 chicken breasts, boneless and cubed
- 20 slices of almond butter lettuce leaves
- ¾ cup cherry tomatoes halved
- 1 avocado, chopped
- ¼ cup green onions, diced
- ½ cup ranch dressing
- ¾ cup hot sauce

How To:

1. Take a bowl and add chicken cubes and sauce , mix.

2. Place within the fridge and let it marinate for half-hour .

3. Preheat your oven to 400 degrees F.

4. Place coated chicken on a cookie pan and bake for 9 minutes.

5. Assemble lettuce serving cups with equal amounts of lettuce, green onions, tomatoes, ranch dressing, and cubed chicken.

6.   Serve and enjoy!

Nutrition (Per Serving)

Calories: 106

Fat: 6g

Net Carbohydrates: 2g

Protein: 5g

Crazy Japanese Potato and Beef Croquettes

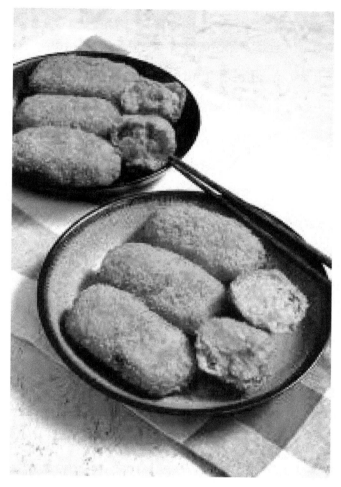

Serving: 10

Prep Time: 10 minute

Cook Time: 20 minutes

Ingredients:

- 3 medium russet potatoes, peeled and chopped
- 1 tablespoon almond butter
- 1 tablespoon vegetable oil
- 3 onions, diced
- ¾ pound ground beef
- 4 teaspoons light coconut aminos
- All-purpose flour for coating
- 2 eggs, beaten
- Panko bread crumbs for coating
- ½ cup oil, frying

How To:

1.   Take a saucepan and place it over medium-high heat; add potatoes and sunflower seeds water, boil for 16 minutes.

2.   Remove water and put potatoes in another bowl, add almond butter and mash the potatoes.

3.   Take a frypan and place it over medium heat, add 1 tablespoon oil and let it heat up.

4.   Add onions and fry until tender.

5.   Add coconut aminos to beef to onions.

6.   Keep frying until beef is browned.

7. Mix the meat with the potatoes evenly.

8. Take another frypan and place it over medium heat; add half a cup of oil.

9. Form croquettes using the potato mixture and coat them with flour, then eggs and eventually breadcrumbs.

10. Fry patties until golden on all sides.

11. Enjoy!

Nutrition (Per Serving)

Calories: 239

Fat: 4g

Carbohydrates: 20g

Protein: 10g

Spicy Chili Crackers

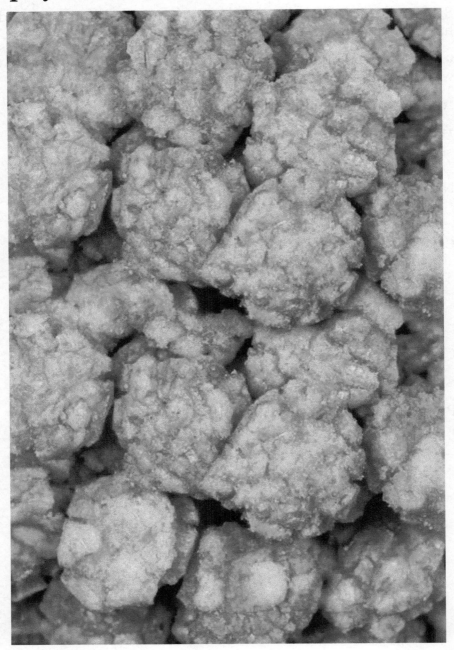

Serving: 30 crackers

Prep Time: 15 minutes

Cooking Time: 60 minutes

Ingredients:

- ¾ cup almond flour
- ¼ cup coconut four
- ¼ cup coconut flour
- ½ teaspoon paprika
- ½ teaspoon cumin
- 1 ½ teaspoons chili pepper spice
- 1 teaspoon onion powder
- ½ teaspoon sunflower seeds
- 1 whole egg
- ¼ cup unsalted almond butter

How To:

1.   Preheat your oven to 350 degrees F.

2.   Line a baking sheet with parchment paper and keep it on the side.

3.   Add ingredients to your kitchen appliance and pulse until you've got a pleasant dough.

4.   Divide dough into two equal parts.

5.   Place one ball on a sheet of parchment paper and canopy with another sheet; roll it out.

6.   dig crackers and repeat with the opposite ball.

7.   Transfer the prepped dough to a baking tray and bake for 8-10 minutes.

8.   Remove from oven and serve.

9.   Enjoy!

Nutrition (Per Serving)

Total Carbs: 2.8g

Fiber: 1g

Protein: 1.6g

Fat: 4.1g

Mushroom and Olive "Mediterranean" Steak

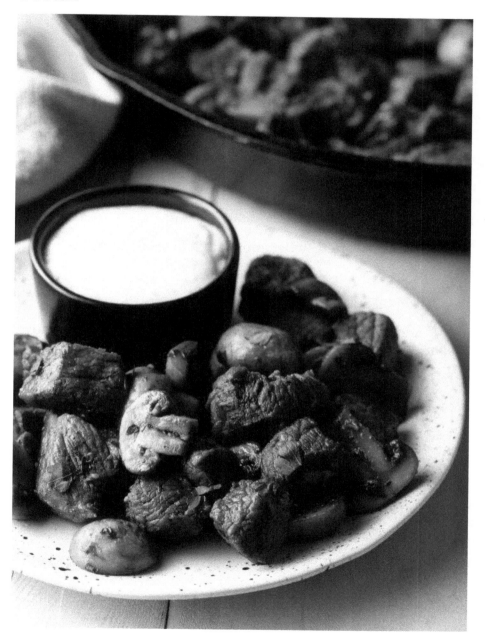

Serving: 2

Prep Time: 10 minutes

Cook Time: 14 minutes

Ingredients:

How To:

Take an outsized sized skillet and place it over medium-high heat.

1.   Add oil and let it heat up.

2.   Add beef and cook until each side are browned, remove beef and drain fat.

3.   Add the remainder of the oil to the skillet and warmth .

4.   Add onions, garlic and cook for 2-3 minutes.

5.   Stir well.

6.   Add mushrooms, olives and cook until the mushrooms are thoroughly done.

7.   Return the meat to the skillet and reduce heat to medium.

8.   Cook for 3-4 minutes (covered).

9.   Stir in parsley.

10.   Serve and enjoy!

Nutrition (Per Serving)

Calories: 386

Fat: 30g

Carbohydrates: 11g

Protein: 21g

Hearty Chicken Fried Rice

Serving: 4

Prep Time: 10 minutes

Cook Time: 12 minutes

Ingredients:

- 1 teaspoon olive oil
- 4 large egg whites
- 1 onion, chopped
- 2 garlic cloves, minced
- 12 ounces skinless chicken breasts, boneless, cut into ½ inch cubes
- ½ cup carrots, chopped
- ½ cup frozen green peas
- 2 cups long grain brown rice, cooked
- 3 tablespoons soy sauce, low sodium

How To:

1.   Coat skillet with oil, place it over medium-high heat.

2.   Add egg whites and cook until scrambled .

3.   Sauté onion, garlic and chicken breasts for six minutes.

4.   Add carrots, peas and keep cooking for 3 minutes.

5.   Stir in rice, season with soy .

6.   Add cooked egg whites, stir for 3 minutes.

7.   Enjoy!

Nutrition (Per Serving)

Calories: 353

Fat: 11g

Carbohydrates: 30g

Protein: 23g

Veggie Quesadillas with Cilantro Yogurt Dip

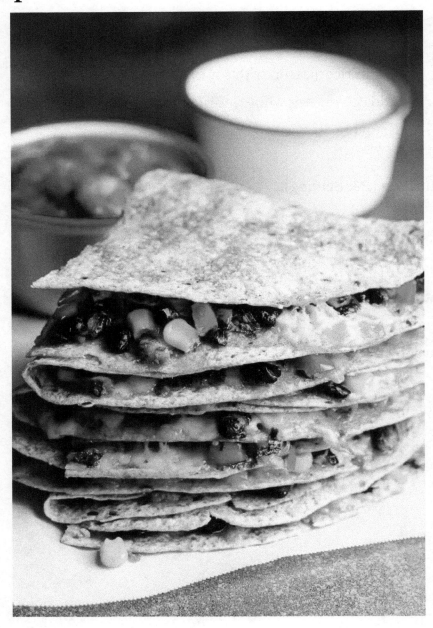

Ingredients

- 1 cup beans, black or pinto
- 2 Tablespoons cilantro, chopped
- ½ bell pepper, finely chopped
- ½ cup corn kernels
- 1 cup low-fat shredded cheese
- Six soft corn tortillas
- One medium carrot, shredded
- ½ jalapeno pepper, finely minced (optional)
- CILANTRO YOGURT DIP
- 1 cup plain nonfat yogurt
- 2 Tablespoons cilantro, finely chopped
- Juice from ½ of a lime

Instructions

1. Preheat large skillet over low heat.

2. Line up three tortillas. Spread cheese, corn, beans, cilantro, shredded carrots, and peppers over the tortillas.

3. Cover all sides with a 2nd tortilla.

4. Place a tortilla on a dry plate and warmth until cheese is melted and tortilla is slightly golden after 3 minutes.

5. Flip and cook another side until golden, about 1 minute.

6.   Inside a small bowl, mix the nonfat yogurt, cilantro, and juice.

7.   Cut each quesadilla into four wedges (12 wedges total) and serve three wedges per person with about ¼ cup of the dip.

8.   Refrigerate leftovers within 2 hours.

Yogurt with Almonds & Honey

Ingredients

- Non-fat greek yoghurt-Nonfat, plain-16 oz-453 grams
- Almonds-Nuts, raw-1/4 cup, whole-35.8 grams
- Honey-2 tsp-14.1 grams

Directions

Rough-chop almonds and blend into yogurt and honey. Enjoy!

Nutrition

Calories 517 Carbs 36g Fat 20g Protein 54g Fiber 5g Net carbs 31g
Sodium 164mg Cholesterol 23mg

Quick Buffalo Chicken Salad

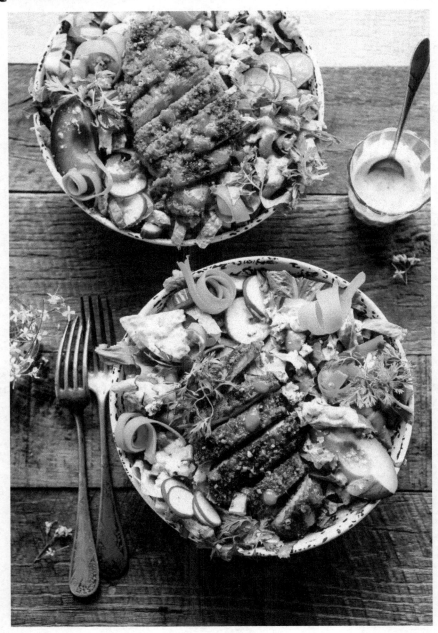

Ingredients

- Pepper or hot sauce-Ready-to-serve-4 tbsp-57.6 grams
- Canned chicken-No broth-1 cup-205 grams
- Spinach-Raw-2 cup-60 grams
- Tomatoes-Green, raw-Two medium-246 grams

Directions

Mix hot sauce with chicken. Spread spinach and tomatoes on the top. Toss together and enjoy it!

Nutrition

Calorie 456 Carbs 18g Fat 18g Protein 57g Fiber 4g Net carbs 13g Sodium 2590mg Cholesterol 103mg

All American Tuna

Ingredients

- Tuna-Fish, light, canned in water, drained solids-Two can-330 grams
- Light mayonnaise-Salad dressing, light-
- 2 tbsp-30 grams Celery-Cooked, boiled, drained, without a salt-1/4 cup, diced-37.5 grams
- Pickles-Cucumber, dill or kosher dill-One large (4" long)-135 grams
- Wheat bread-Two slice-50 grams

Directions

1. Mix all ingredients in a bowl.

2. Serve with bread.

Nutrition

Calories 512 Carbs 32g Fat 12g Protein 71g Fiber 4g Net carbs 28g Sodium 2443mg Cholesterol 124mg

Chicken Salsa

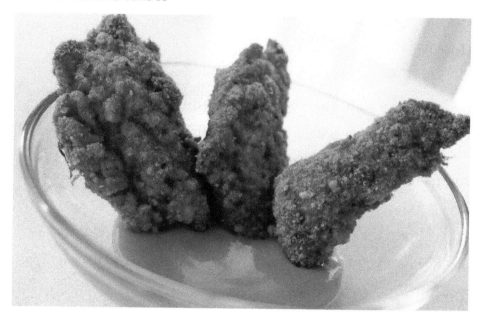

Serving: 1

Prep Time: 4 minutes

Cook Time: 14 minutes

Ingredients:

- 2 chicken breasts
- 1 cup salsa
- 1 taco seasoning mix
- 1 cup plain Greek Yogurt

- ½ cup of kite ricottta/cashew cheese, cubed

How To:

1.   Take a skillet and place over medium heat.

2.   Add pigeon breast , ½ cup of salsa and taco seasoning.

3.   Mix well and cook for 12-15 minutes until the chicken is completed .

4.   Take the back off and cube them.

5.   Place the cubes on toothpick and top with cheddar.

6.   Place yogurt and remaining salsa in cups and use as dips.

7. Enjoy!

Nutrition (Per Serving)

Calories: 359

Fat: 14g

Net Carbohydrates: 14g

Protein: 43g

Healthy Mediterranean Lamb Chops

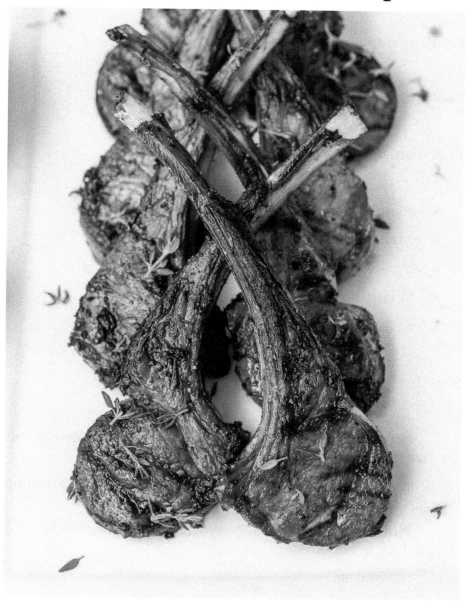

Serving: 4

Prep Time: 10 minutes

Cook Time: 10 minutes

Ingredients:

- 4 lamb shoulder chops, 8 ounces each
- 2 tablespoons Dijon mustard
- 2 tablespoons Balsamic vinegar
- ½ cup olive oil
- 2 tablespoons shredded fresh basil

How To:

1.   Pat your lamb chop dry employing a kitchen towel and arrange them on a shallow glass baking dish.

2.   Take a bowl and a whisk in Dijon mustard, balsamic vinegar, pepper and blend them well.

3.   Whisk within the oil very slowly into the marinade until the mixture is smooth

4.   Stir in basil.

5.   Pour the marinade over the lamb chops and stir to coat each side well.

6.   Cover the chops and permit them to marinate for 1-4 hours (chilled).

7.   Take the chops out and leave them for half-hour to permit the temperature to succeed in a traditional level.

8.   Pre-heat your grill to medium heat and add oil to the grate.

9.   Grill the lamb chops for 5-10 minutes per side until each side are browned.

10.   Once the middle reads 145 degrees F, the chops are ready, serve and enjoy!

Nutrition (Per Serving)

Calories: 521

Fat: 45g

Carbohydrates: 3.5g

Protein: 22g

Amazing Sesame Breadsticks

Serving: 5 breadsticks

Prep Time: 10 minutes

Cooking Time: 20 minutes

Ingredients:

- 1 egg white
- 2 tablespoons almond flour
- 1 teaspoon Himalayan pink sunflower seeds
- 1 tablespoon extra-virgin olive oil
- ½ teaspoon sesame seeds

How To:

1.   Pre-heat your oven to 320 degrees F.

2.   Line a baking sheet with parchment paper and keep it on the side.

3.   Take a bowl and whisk in egg whites, add flour and half sunflower seeds and vegetable oil .

4.   Knead until you've got a smooth dough.

5.   Divide into 4 pieces and roll into breadsticks.

6.   Place on prepared sheet and brush with vegetable oil , sprinkle sesame seeds and remaining sunflower seeds.

7.   Bake for 20 minutes.

8.   Serve and enjoy!

Nutrition (Per Serving)

Total Carbs: 1.1g

Fiber: 1g

Protein: 1.6g

Fat: 5g

Brown Butter Duck Breast

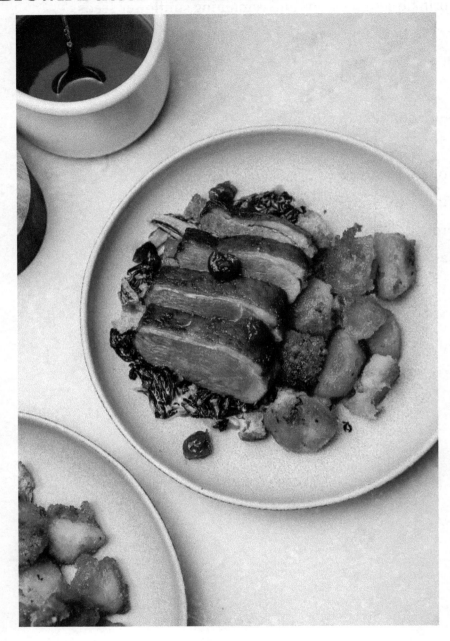

Serving: 3

Prep Time: 5 minutes

Cook Time: 25 minutes

Ingredients:

- 1 whole 6 ounce duck breast, skin on
- Pepper to taste
- 1 head radicchio, 4 ounces, core removed
- ¼ cup unsalted utter
- 6 fresh sage leaves, sliced

How To:

1.   Pre-heat your oven to 400 degree F.

2.   Pat duck breast dry with towel .

3.   Season with pepper.

4.   Place duck breast in skillet and place it over medium heat, sear for 3-4 minutes all sides

5.   Turn breast over and transfer skillet to oven.

6.   Roast for 10 minutes (uncovered).

7.   Cut radicchio in half.

8.   Remove and discard the woody white core and thinly slice the leaves.

9.   Keep them on the side.

10.   Remove skillet from oven.

11.   Transfer duck breast, fat side up to chopping board and let it rest.12.   Re-heat your skillet over medium heat.

13. Add unsalted butter, sage and cook for 3-4 minutes.

14.   Cut duck into 6 equal slices.

15.   Divide radicchio between 2 plates, top with slices of duck breast and drizzle browned butter and sage.

16.   Enjoy!

Nutrition (Per Serving)

Calories: 393

Fat: 33g

Carbohydrates: 2g

Protein: 22g

Generous Garlic Bread Stick

Serving: 8 breadsticks

Prep Time: 15 minutes

Cooking Time: 15 minutes

Ingredients:

- ¼ cup almond butter, softened
- 1 teaspoon garlic powder
- 2 cups almond flour
- ½ tablespoon baking powder
- 1 tablespoon Psyllium husk powder
- ¼ teaspoon sunflower seeds
- 3 tablespoons almond butter, melted
- 1 egg
- ¼ cup boiling water

How To:

1.   Pre-heat your oven to 400 degrees F.

2.   Line baking sheet with parchment paper and keep it on the side.

3.   Beat almond butter with garlic powder and keep it on the side.

4.   Add almond flour, leaven , husk, sunflower seeds during a bowl and blend in almond butter and egg, mix well.

5.   Pour boiling water within the mix and stir until you've got a pleasant dough.

6.   Divide the dough into 8 balls and roll into breadsticks.

7.   Place on baking sheet and bake for quarter-hour .

8.   Brush each persist with garlic almond butter and bake for five minutes more.

9.   Serve and enjoy!

Nutrition (Per Serving)

Total Carbs: 7g

Fiber: 2g

Protein: 7g

Fat: 24g

Chicken & Goat Cheese Skillet

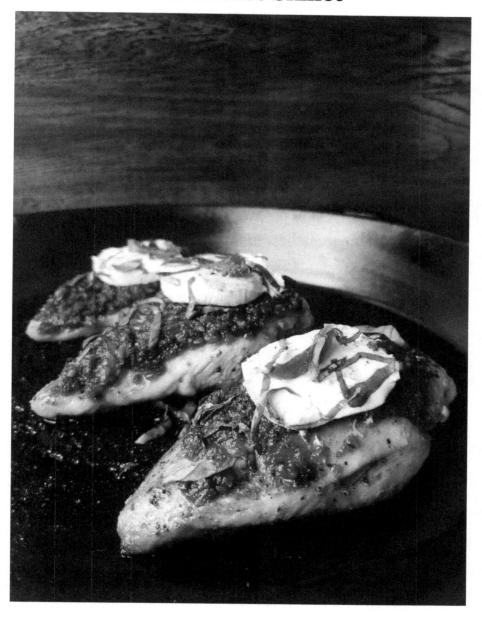

Ingredients

- 1/2 pound of boneless skinless chicken breasts, cut into 1-inch pieces
- 1/4 teaspoon salt
- 1/8 teaspoon pepper
- Two teaspoons olive oil
- 1 cup sliced fresh asparagus (1-inch pieces)
- One garlic clove, minced
- Three plum tomatoes, chopped
- Three tablespoons 2% milk
- Two tablespoons herbed fresh goat cheese, crumbled
- Hot cooked rice or pasta
- Additional goat cheese, optional

Directions

1.   Toss chicken with salt and pepper. Heat oil at medium heat; saute chicken until not pink, 4-6 minutes.Remove from pan; keep warm.

2.   Add asparagus to skillet; cook and blend at medium-high heat 1 minute. Add garlic; cook and stir 30 seconds. Stirin tomatoes, milk, and two tablespoons cheese; cook, covered, over medium heat until cheese begins to melt, 2-3 minutes. Stir in chicken. Serve with rice. If desired, top with additional cheese.

Nutrition

251 calories, 11g fat, 74mg cholesterol, 447mg sodium, 8g carbohydrate (5g sugars, 3g fiber), 29g protein. Diabetic Exchanges: 4 lean meat, two fat, one vegetable.

Green Curry Salmon with Green Beans

Ingredients

- Four salmon fillets (4 ounces each)
- 1 cup light coconut milk
- Two tablespoons green curry paste
- 1 cup uncooked instant brown rice
- 1 cup reduced-sodium chicken broth
- 1/8 teaspoon pepper
- 3/4 pound fresh green beans, trimmed
- One teaspoon sesame oil
- One teaspoon sesame seeds, toasted
- Lime wedges

Directions

1. Preheat oven to 400°. Place salmon in an 8-in. Square baking dish. Mix together coconut milk and curry paste; pour over salmon. Bake, uncovered, till fish simply starts offevolved to flake effortlessly with a fork, 15-20 minutes.

2. Meanwhile, during a small saucepan, integrate rice, broth and pepper; convey to a boil. Reduce warmth; simmer, covered, 5 minutes. Remove from heat; let stand five minutes.

3.   In a big saucepan, area steamer basket over 1 in. Of water. Place inexperienced beans inside the basket; convey water to a boil. Reduce heat to take care of a simmer; steam, covered, till beans are crisp-tender, 7-10 minutes. Toss with vegetable oil and sesame seeds.

4.   Serve salmon with rice, beans and lime wedges. Spoon coconut sauce over the salmon.

Nutrition Facts

366 calories, 17g fat (5g saturated fat), 57mg cholesterol, 340mg sodium, 29g carbohydrate (5g sugars, 4g fibre), 24g protein.

Chicken Veggie Packets

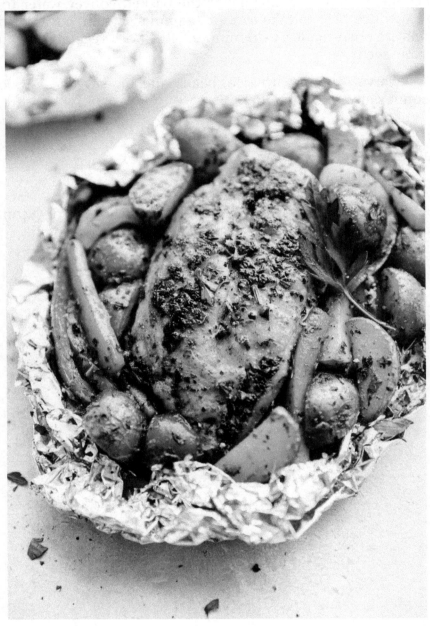

Ingredients

- Four boneless and skinless chicken breast halves (4 ounces each)
- 1/2 pound sliced fresh mushrooms
- 1-1/2 cups fresh baby carrots
- 1 cup pearl onions
- 1/2 cup julienned sweet red pepper
- 1/4 teaspoon pepper
- Three teaspoons minced fresh thyme
- 1/2 teaspoon salt, optional
- Lemon wedges, optional

Directions

1.   Flatten bird breasts to 1/2-in. Thickness; vicinity every on a touch of industrial quality foil (about 12 in. Square). Layer the mushrooms, carrots, onions and pink pepper over bird; sprinkle with pepper, thyme and salt if desired.

2.   Fold foil around hen and greens and seal tightly. Place on a baking sheet. Bake at 375° for a half-hour or until chook juices run clear. If desired, serve with lemon wedges.

Nutrition Facts

175 calories, 3g fat (1g saturated fat), 63mg cholesterol, 100mg sodium, 11g carbohydrate (6g sugars, 2g fibre), 25g protein.

Sweet Onion & Sausage Spaghetti

Ingredients

- 6 ounces uncooked whole-wheat spaghetti
- 3/4 pound Italian turkey sausage links, casings removed
- Two teaspoons olive oil
- One sweet onion, thinly sliced
- 1-pint cherry tomatoes halved
- One and a half cup of fresh basil leaves (sliced)
- 1/2 cup half-and-half cream
- Shaved Parmesan cheese, optional

Directions

1.   Cook spaghetti consistent with directions given. At an equivalent time, during a large nonstick skillet over medium heat, cook sausage in oil for five minutes. Add onion; bake 8-10 minutes longer or until meat is not any longer pink and onion is tender.

2.   Stir in tomatoes and basil; heat through. Add cream; bring back a boil. Drain spaghetti; toss with sausage mixture. Garnish with cheese if desired.

Nutrition Facts

334 calories, 12g fat (4g saturated fat), 46mg cholesterol, 378mg sodium, 41g carbohydrate (8g sugars, 6g fibre), 17g protein.

Beef and Blue Cheese Penne with Pesto

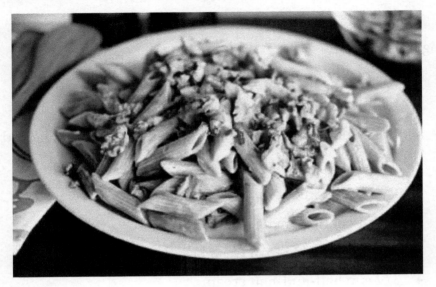

Ingredients

- 2 cups uncooked whole wheat penne pasta
- Two beef tenderloin steaks (6 ounces each)
- 1/4 teaspoon salt
- 1/4 teaspoon pepper
- 5 ounces of fresh baby spinach (about 6 cups), coarsely chopped
- 2 cups grape tomatoes, halved
- 1/3 cup prepared pesto
- 1/4 cup chopped walnuts
- 1/4 cup crumbled Gorgonzola cheese

Directions

1.   Cook pasta consistent with package directions.

2.   Meanwhile, sprinkle steaks with salt and pepper. Grill steaks, covered, over medium heat. Heat for 5-7 mins on all sides or until meat reaches desired doneness.

3.   Drain pasta; transfer to an outsized bowl. Add spinach, tomatoes, pesto and walnuts; toss to coat. Cut steak into thin slices. Serve pasta mixture with beef; sprinkle with cheese.

Nutrition Facts

532 calories, 22g fat (6g saturated fat), 50mg cholesterol, 434mg sodium, 49g carbohydrate (3g sugars, 9g fibre), 35g protein.

Asparagus Turkey Stir-Fry

Ingredients

- Two teaspoons cornstarch
- 1/4 cup chicken broth
- One tablespoon lemon juice
- One teaspoon soy sauce
- 1 pound of turkey breast tenderloins, cut into 1/2-inch strips
- One garlic clove, minced
- Two tablespoons canola oil, divided
- 1 pound of asparagus, cut into 1-1/2-inch pieces
- One jar (2 ounces) sliced pimientos, drained

Instructions

1.   In a little bowl, mix the cornstarch, broth, juice and soy until smooth; put aside . during a large skillet orwok, stir-fry turkey and garlic in 1 tablespoon oil until meat is not any longer pink; remove and keep warm.

2.   Stir-fry asparagus in remaining oil until crisp-tender. Add pimientos. Stir the mixture and increase the pan; cook andstir for 1 minute or until thickened. Return turkey to the pan; heat through.

Nutrition Facts

205 calories, 9g fat (1g saturated fat), 56mg cholesterol, 204mg sodium, 5g carbohydrate (1g sugars, 1g fibre), 28g protein.

Awesome Cabbage Soup

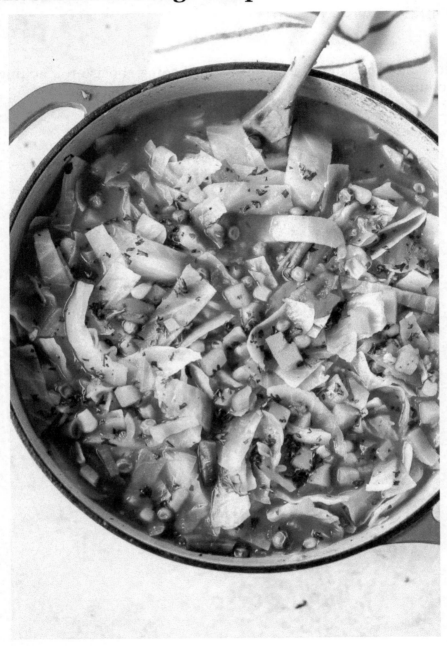

Serving: 3

Prep Time: 7 minutes

Cook Time: 25 minutes

Ingredients:

- 3 cups non-fat beef stock
- 2 garlic cloves, minced
- 1 tablespoon tomato paste
- 2 cups cabbage, chopped
- ½ yellow onion
- ½ cup carrot, chopped
- ½ cup green beans
- ½ cup zucchini, chopped
- ½ teaspoon basil
- ½ teaspoon oregano
- Sunflower seeds and pepper as needed

How To:

1.   Grease a pot with non-stick cooking spray.

2.   Place it over medium heat and permit the oil to heat up.

3.   Add onions, carrots, and garlic and sauté for five minutes.

4.   Add broth, ingredient , green beans, cabbage, basil, oregano, sunflower seeds, and pepper.

5.   Bring the entire mix to a boil and reduce the warmth , simmer for 5-10 minutes until all veggies are tender.

6.   Add zucchini and simmer for five minutes more.

7.   Sever hot and enjoy!

Nutrition (Per Serving)

Calories: 22

Fat: 0g

Carbohydrates: 5g

Protein: 1g

Ginger Zucchini Avocado Soup

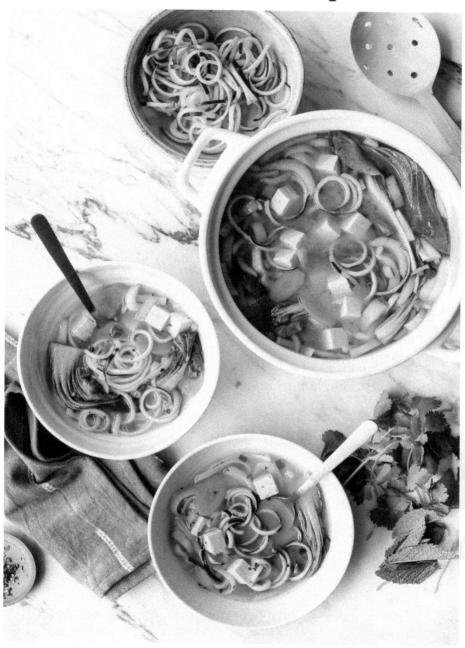

Serving: 3

Prep Time: 7 minutes

Cook Time: 25 minutes

Ingredients:

- 1 red bell pepper, chopped
- 1 big avocado
- 1 teaspoon ginger, grated
- Pepper as needed
- 2 tablespoons avocado oil
- 4 scallions, chopped
- 1 tablespoon lemon juice
- 29 ounces vegetable stock
- 1 garlic clove, minced
- 2 zucchini, chopped
- 1 cup water

How To:

1.   Take a pan and place over medium heat, add onion and fry for 3 minutes.

2.   Stir in ginger, garlic and cook for 1 minute.

3.   Mix in seasoning, zucchini stock, water and boil for 10 minutes.

4.   Remove soup from fire and let it sit, blend in avocado and blend using an immersion blender.

5.   Heat over low heat for a short time .

6.   Adjust your seasoning and add juice , bell pepper.

7.   Serve and enjoy!

Nutrition (Per Serving)

Calories: 155

Fat: 11g

Carbohydrates: 10g

Protein: 7g

Greek Lemon and Chicken Soup

Serving: 4

Prep Time: 15 minutes

Cook Time: 30 minutes

Ingredients:

- 2 cups cooked chicken, chopped
- 2 medium carrots, chopped
- ½ cup onion, chopped ¼ cup lemon juice
- 1 clove garlic, minced
- 1 can cream of chicken soup, fat-free and low sodium
- 2 cans chicken broth, fat-free
- ¼ teaspoon ground black pepper
- 2/3 cup long-grain rice
- 2 tablespoons parsley, snipped

How To:

1.   Add all of the listed ingredients to a pot (except rice and parsley).

2.   Season with sunflower seeds and pepper.

3.   Bring the combination to a overboil medium-high heat.

4.   Stir in rice and set heat to medium.

5.   Simmer for 20 minutes until rice is tender.

6.   Garnish parsley and enjoy!

Nutrition (Per Serving)

Calories: 582

Fat: 33g

Carbohydrates: 35g

Protein: 32g

Morning Peach

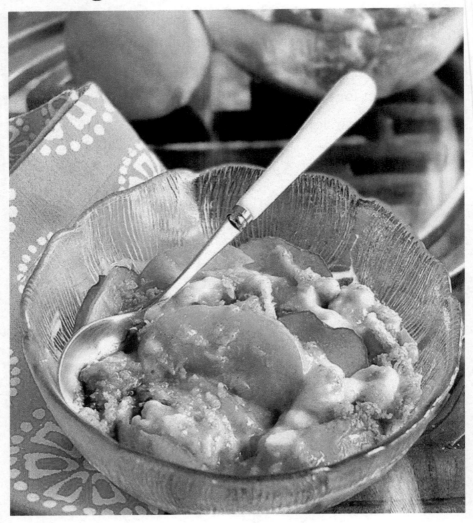

Serving: 4

Prep Time: 10 minutes

Cook Time: 5 minutes

Ingredients:

- 6 small peaches, cored and cut into wedges
- ¼ cup coconut sugar
- 2 tablespoons almond butter
- ¼ teaspoon almond extract

How To:

1.   Take a little pan and add peaches, sugar, butter and flavor.

2.   Toss well.

3.   Cook over medium-high heat for five minutes, divide the combination into bowls and serve.

4.   Enjoy!

Nutrition (Per Serving)

Calories: 198

Fat: 2g

Carbohydrates: 11g

Protein: 8g

Garlic and Pumpkin Soup

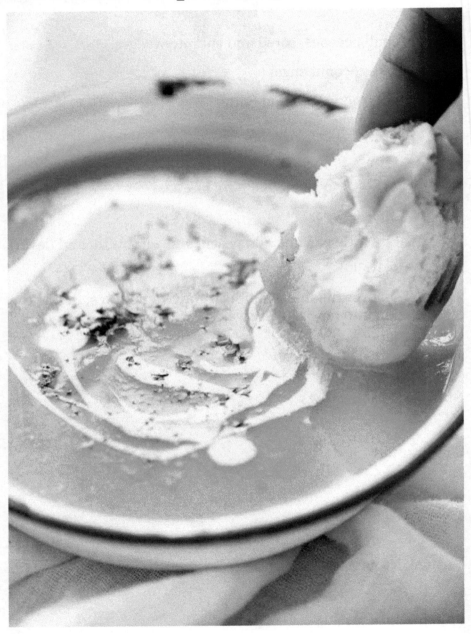

Serving: 4

Prep Time: 10 minutes

Cook Time: 5 hours

Ingredients:

- 1-pound pumpkin chunks
- 1 onion, diced
- 2 cups vegetable stock
- 1 2/3 cups coconut cream
- ½ stick almond butter
- 1 teaspoon garlic, crushed
- 1 teaspoon ginger, crushed
- Pepper to taste

How To:

1. Add all the ingredients into your Slow Cooker.
2. Cook for 4-6 hours on high.
3. Puree the soup by using an immersion blender.
4. Serve and enjoy!

Nutrition (Per Serving)

Calories: 235

Fat: 21g

Carbohydrates: 11g

Protein: 2g

Lightning Source UK Ltd.
Milton Keynes UK
UKHW020704130521
383649UK00005B/119